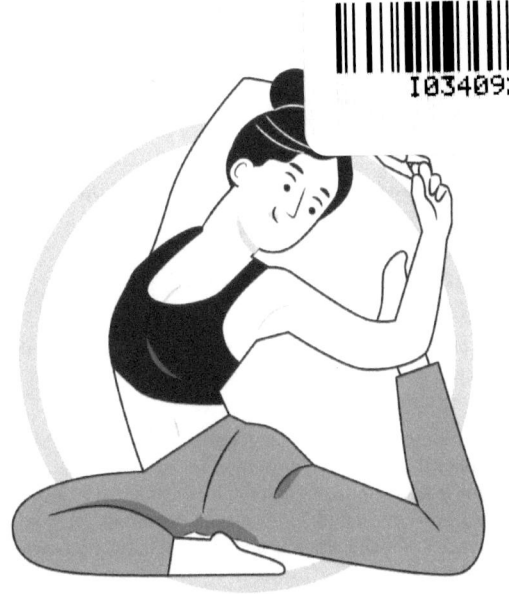

POSITIVE AFFIRMATIONS AND ACTIONS FOR

Health

USE YOUR SELF CARE DAILY RITUALS TO LEARN TO LOVE YOURSELF, CREATE HAPPINESS, IMPROVE YOUR CONFIDENCE & BUILD INNER STRENGTH

🐢 Turtle Publishing

Published by Turtle Publishing
All rights reserved.

Printed on demand in Australia, United States and United Kingdom.

Written & designed by Kathy Shanks
© Kathy Shanks 2021
Illustrations by Freepik Storyset & Turtle Publishing

No part of this publication may be reproduced, stored in a retrieval system, or transmitted in any form or by any means, electronic, mechanical, photocopying, recording or otherwise, without the prior written permission of the author.

Under no circumstances will any blame or legal responsibility be held against the publisher, or author, for any damages, reparation, or monetary loss due to the information contained within this book including, but not limited to — errors, omissions, or inaccuracies. Either directly or indirectly. You are responsible for your own choices, actions, and results.

Legal Notice: This book is copyright protected. This book is only for personal use. You cannot amend, distribute, sell, use, quote or paraphrase any part, or the content within this book, without the consent of the author or publisher.

Disclaimer: Please note the information contained within this document is for educational and entertainment purposes only. All effort has been executed to present accurate, up to date, and reliable, complete information. No warranties of any kind are declared or implied. Readers acknowledge that the author is not engaging in the rendering of legal, financial, medical or professional advice. The content within this book has been derived from various sources. Please consult a licensed professional before attempting any techniques outlined in this book.

🐢 TurtlePublishing

SPECIAL BONUS
FREE BOOKS

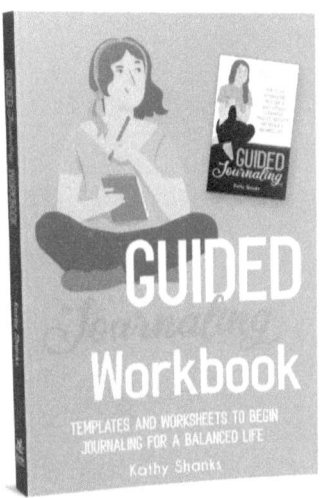 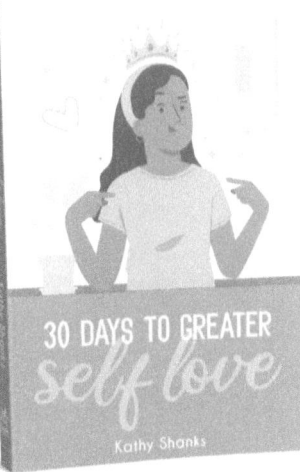

FREE Workbook to begin an intentional journaling practice.

FREE 30 Days to Greater Self Love Program

Get FREE unlimited access to these AND all of my new books by joining our fan base!

SCAN WITH YOUR CAMERA OR GO TO
bit.ly/AffGifts

How to use this book

On the left-hand pages are affirmations. On the right-hand pages are actions for you to take for your physical, emotional and mental health.

You may like to work through this book one page per day, or perhaps you'd like to trust divine guidance. Hold this book close to your heart or navel, close your eyes, take three gentle breaths, and as you breathe out on the third breath, open the book. We trust that you will be guided to the page you need the most.

Introduction

Whether you're aware of it or not, your health plays a massive part in your life. In fact, it may very well be at the centre of it all. Working towards your goals, being a blessing to others, enjoying your hobbies and the things you do for fun, and simply being a productive member of society... none of it would be possible if you were unhealthy.

But, what does being healthy really mean? What comes to mind when you think of "health?" Perhaps living an active lifestyle and eating food that's good for you? Or, maybe hitting your ideal weight and getting the body you've always wanted?

In a society that can be hyper-fixated on looks, the physical aspect of health is frequently grossly oversimplified. It is usually whittled down to the bare minimum of an absence of illness and often, maintaining a certain weight and having a 'fit' body.

However, the reality is that looking good is primarily just a sign or 'side effect' of physical health—of your body's systems being in peak condition and all its processes functioning smoothly. While exercise and balanced nutrition are definitely important in achieving and maintaining this, there are so many other factors. These include getting enough good quality sleep and adequate rest, proper hydration, and access to medical support (as needed).

Not only is the idea of physical health limited to such a narrow definition, but even worse, there's also a tendency to disregard all the other aspects of health. While wanting to maintain a particular physique is valid and physical fitness can indeed be an essential component of health, there is so much more to it than just that.

Being healthy also includes mental, emotional, social, and even spiritual wellbeing. All of these are interconnected, and being truly healthy entails understanding and tending to yourself holistically.

First off, mental health is how you process and interpret information and the world around you, including making decisions and managing stress. The term is often used interchangeably with emotional health, but while these certainly overlap, they are not one and the same. As mental health deals with the brain and its functions, you can almost think of it as emotional health's 'physical' counterpart.

On the other hand, emotional health has to do with how you manage feelings. It absolutely doesn't mean always being positive and happy—rather, it's about the ability to deal even with negative emotions. Given that, self-awareness and authenticity play a huge role in emotional health, as these serve as the foundation for developing coping skills to navigate different contexts and situations.

Both mental and emotional dimensions come into play when it comes to our social health or the ability to form meaningful relationships, whether with family, friends, a significant other, or the community at large.

Lastly, the spiritual aspect is possibly one of the most overlooked components of health. Perhaps it's no surprise, as it's not the easiest concept to fit into a singular, neat definition. For many, this could be their practice of faith. For others, it's not necessarily religious, and more a matter of how they fit into the 'big picture'—having that sense of connectedness and purpose.

With this deeper, broader picture of health, it can no doubt be even more daunting to commit to working on your wellbeing. As with anything worthwhile, though, remember that achieving health takes time—it's a process. It's about making one small change at a time, building habits that serve you to replace those that do not.

Along with small-yet-impactful actions, an affirmation practice can be of great help when it comes to health and wellness. Not only does it channel healing energy and strength towards the areas in your life that need it the most, but because your mind, body, heart, and soul are all interconnected, it also empowers you to set positive change in motion across all aspects. Repeating thought patterns that reinforce certain behaviours and beliefs actually makes it easier for you to make healthier choices in your life.

Affirmations also serve as reinforcements for self-care and self-love, two of the most powerful tools in your health and wellbeing journey. The ability to listen to your body and love yourself through it all is so incredibly important.

Each picture of health—and the path to it—is unique. Your goals, milestones, and pace are all wonderfully, gloriously different from everybody else's... and that is beyond okay. No matter where you are on this journey, you deserve to enjoy life and cherish yourself every step of the way.

"Wellness is the complete integration of body, mind, and spirit – the realization that everything we do, think, feel, and believe has an effect on our state of well-being."

- Greg Anderson

AFFIRMATIONS

I love who I am, and I'm excited about who I am becoming.

ACTIONS

Begin your day with some energising morning stretches.

AFFIRMATIONS

I am strong and
filled with life.

ACTIONS

Hydrate! Always make sure you are getting enough water throughout the day.

AFFIRMATIONS

Energy flows
through
my body
effortlessly.

ACTIONS

Create a bedtime ritual that helps you wind down and relax. It doesn't have to take long or be complicated—it can be as simple as having a cup of tea or listening to a soothing song.

AFFIRMATIONS

My body serves me well.

ACTIONS

When you find yourself stressed or anxious, take a moment to pause, close your eyes, and take 10 long, deep breaths.

AFFIRMATIONS

I honour the shape of my body.

ACTIONS

Try to learn about and get a deeper understanding of what you put on and into your body.

AFFIRMATIONS

I am happy to
be uniquely me.

ACTIONS

Pick some affirmations that really resonate with you, and practice saying these out loud to yourself in front of the mirror each day.

AFFIRMATIONS

I love my body and everything it does for me every day.

ACTIONS

Give yourself at least 10 minutes each day to meditate or practice mindfulness.

AFFIRMATIONS

I am capable of making healthy decisions for my body and mind.

ACTIONS

Start your day with a hearty, balanced breakfast.

AFFIRMATIONS

I deserve to
spend time
and energy
on things that
make me happy.

ACTIONS

List down 10 things you adore about your body.

AFFIRMATIONS

I am at
peace with
all my body's
imperfections.

ACTIONS

Stock your pantry with wholesome, nutritious snacks.

AFFIRMATIONS

I am deeply committed to caring for myself.

ACTIONS

Once a week, treat yourself to something you really, truly enjoy.

AFFIRMATIONS

I am capable of setting healthy boundaries for myself.

ACTIONS

Put on some of your favourite upbeat music, turn it up, and dance!

AFFIRMATIONS

I am allowed to put myself first.

ACTIONS

Get your daily dose of vitamin D—sit out in the sunshine for a bit!

AFFIRMATIONS

I am growing
and changing
in all the ways I
am meant to.

ACTIONS

Learn a new sport with your partner or a friend.

AFFIRMATIONS

I am in control of my wellbeing.

ACTIONS

Do your best to get as much sleep as your body needs. For many, this would be about 7-9 hours nightly.

AFFIRMATIONS

I am nourished in both mind and body.

ACTIONS

Practice listening to what your body is telling you and responding mindfully to its needs.

AFFIRMATIONS

I deserve rest
whenever I
need it.

ACTIONS

It's time to finally get rid of those clothes in the depths of your closet that no longer fit.

AFFIRMATIONS

I am free to move and be active.

ACTIONS

Try out a new delicious, nutritious recipe every week.

AFFIRMATIONS

I have the power to lift myself up.

ACTIONS

Run a luxurious bath with your favourite scent and give yourself as much time as you want to enjoy it.

AFFIRMATIONS

I deserve the best health and a fit body.

ACTIONS

Squeeze in at least 10-15 minutes of exercise every day. It can be as simple as getting your heart rate up with a short walk or doing a few reps of light weights.

AFFIRMATIONS

I honour my
inner power.

ACTIONS

As much as possible, avoid screens and blue light an hour before bed.

AFFIRMATIONS

I am allowed to be proud of my accomplishments and celebrate these.

ACTIONS

Make moisturising a post-shower habit—give yourself a little massage while you're at it!

AFFIRMATIONS

I am aging with grace.

ACTIONS

Try out a weekly 'meatless Monday' or 'whole foods Wednesday.'

AFFIRMATIONS

I release any stress and tension in both my mind and body.

ACTIONS

Bring awareness to your posture, both when sitting and standing.

AFFIRMATIONS

Every part of me is worthy of respect.

ACTIONS

Try to enjoy each of your meals mindfully—as much as possible, avoid working lunches and dinners in front of the telly.

AFFIRMATIONS

I let go of thoughts that do not serve me.

ACTIONS

Write down the best compliment you've ever received.

AFFIRMATIONS

I release any expectations I feel pressured to live up to.

ACTIONS

Pick up some self-massage techniques online, or even treat yourself to a session with a professional masseuse.

AFFIRMATIONS

Every cell in my body is brimming with energy.

ACTIONS

Time for a social media audit—unfollow any accounts or influencers that make you feel bad about yourself or don't add any value to your life.

AFFIRMATIONS

I am proud to be a work in progress.

ACTIONS

Start that inspirational book that you've been meaning to get around to.

AFFIRMATIONS

I am a beautiful person inside and out.

ACTIONS

Do an at-home spa day with a DIY face or hair mask.

AFFIRMATIONS

My body's systems are all functioning in perfect harmony.

ACTIONS

Remember not to get caught up with measurements or numbers on a scale—focus on feeling happier, healthier, and stronger.

AFFIRMATIONS

I am in tune
with my body
and its needs.

ACTIONS

Stretch and strengthen your mind, body, and spirit with some yoga practice.

AFFIRMATIONS

Health and wellness flow to me naturally and in abundance.

ACTIONS

Let go of any guilt when it comes to food.

AFFIRMATIONS

I am filled with grit and determination.

ACTIONS

Start a daily mood tracker on your phone or in your journal.

AFFIRMATIONS

I embrace whatever state of health I am in now.

ACTIONS

If you have a dog, commit to taking them out for a walk at least once a day. If not, you might even want to consider volunteering to walk a friend's or neighbours.

AFFIRMATIONS

It's perfectly
okay to both
work on my
body, and at the
same time, love
it for what it is.

ACTIONS

Whenever possible, choose to take the stairs over the elevator or escalator.

AFFIRMATIONS

I deserve all the happiness in the world.

ACTIONS

How long has it been since you've walked barefoot outdoors, on the grass or at the beach?

AFFIRMATIONS

I rise to every challenge in my own unique way.

ACTIONS

List down 5 things you're capable of that not many people can do.

AFFIRMATIONS

I am proud to be my own cheerleader.

ACTIONS

Make time to hang out with a friend who's fun to be around.

AFFIRMATIONS

Disease, illness, or disability does not define me and what I am capable of.

ACTIONS

Have you ever gone a whole day not thinking about what you look like? Challenge yourself to 24 hours without looking at yourself in the mirror, and take note of how it feels.

AFFIRMATIONS

I am surrounded by people who support my wellbeing.

ACTIONS

Commit to keeping a plant or small garden. Set aside time each day to tend to it and enjoy how it flourishes under your care.

AFFIRMATIONS

I am in control of my own happiness.

ACTIONS

Find and learn a breathing exercise that works for you, and use it whenever you need a little pocket of calm in your day.

AFFIRMATIONS

My body has the remarkable capacity to heal itself.

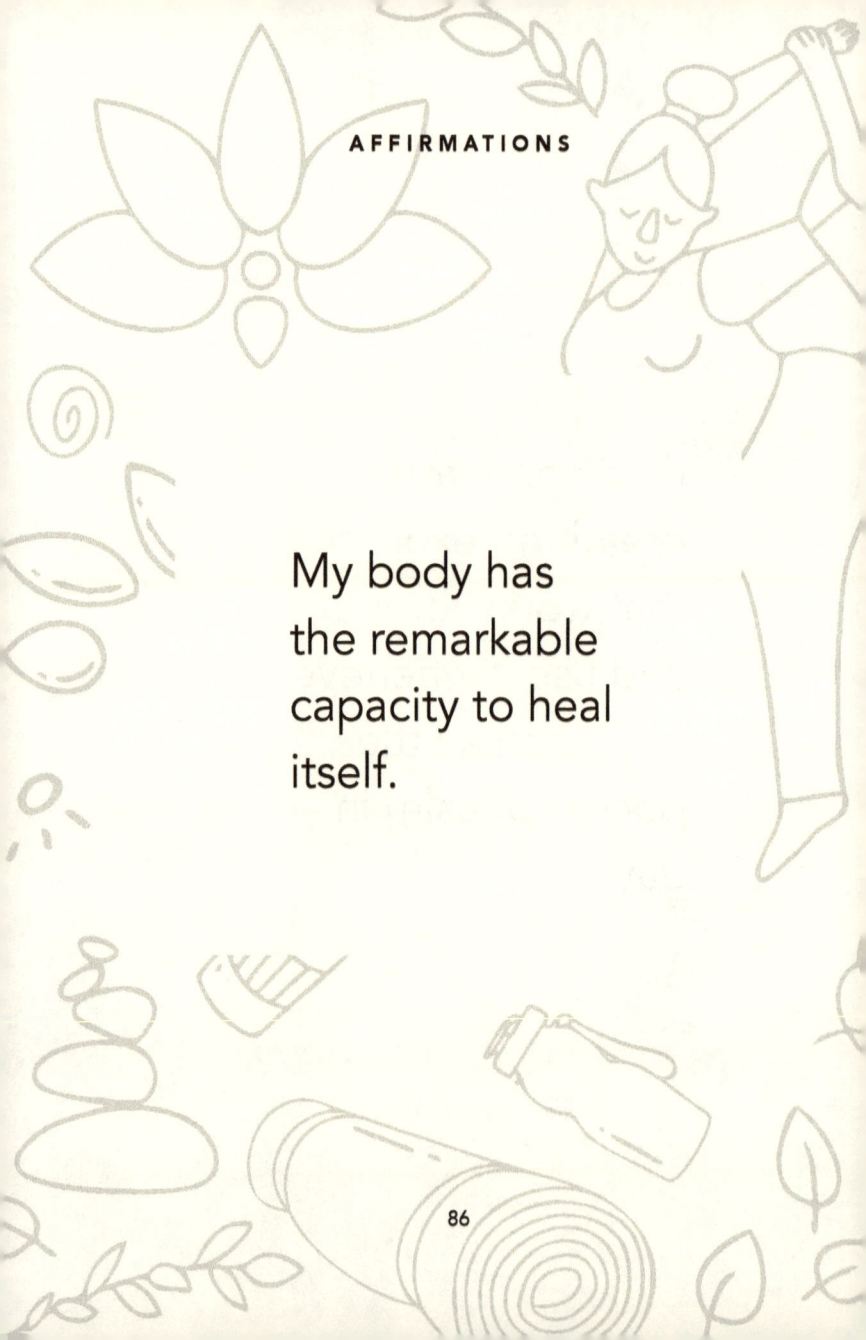

ACTIONS

What makes you feel like your best self? List down everything you can think of.

AFFIRMATIONS

Fear cannot
stand in my way.

ACTIONS

Listen to an uplifting, motivating song. Close your eyes, and enjoy how the music makes you feel.

AFFIRMATIONS

I am patient
with my body.

ACTIONS

Hold a board game night with a group of friends or play a couple of brainteaser puzzles with your family.

AFFIRMATIONS

I am perfectly imperfect.

ACTIONS

Pick up a meditative, calming hobby like knitting or mandala-making.

AFFIRMATIONS

I am capable of so much more than I ever dreamed.

ACTIONS

Watch a feel-good movie or a laugh-out-loud sitcom.

AFFIRMATIONS

I trust in the power of my body.

ACTIONS

Visit your local farmers' market and check out the fresh produce and 'slow' food.

AFFIRMATIONS

My body's journey is uniquely mine.

ACTIONS

When was the last time you saw a sunrise? Pick a day to wake up extra early and enjoy the stillness of dawn.

AFFIRMATIONS

I choose to live in health and vitality.

ACTIONS

List down 5 healthy boundaries or non-negotiables that you would like to start enforcing.

AFFIRMATIONS

Healthy habits are a natural part of me.

ACTIONS

Plan a camping trip or hike!

AFFIRMATIONS

I am allowed to move and grow at my own pace.

ACTIONS

If possible, open all your windows and curtains to let fresh air in.

AFFIRMATIONS

I am focused
and consistent
when it comes
to my health.

ACTIONS

Try a freewriting exercise. No (over)thinking—just put your pen to paper and write from your stream of consciousness.

AFFIRMATIONS

I am always
changing for
the better.

ACTIONS

Put up some blackout curtains to improve the quality of your sleep.

AFFIRMATIONS

I listen to my body and tend to its needs.

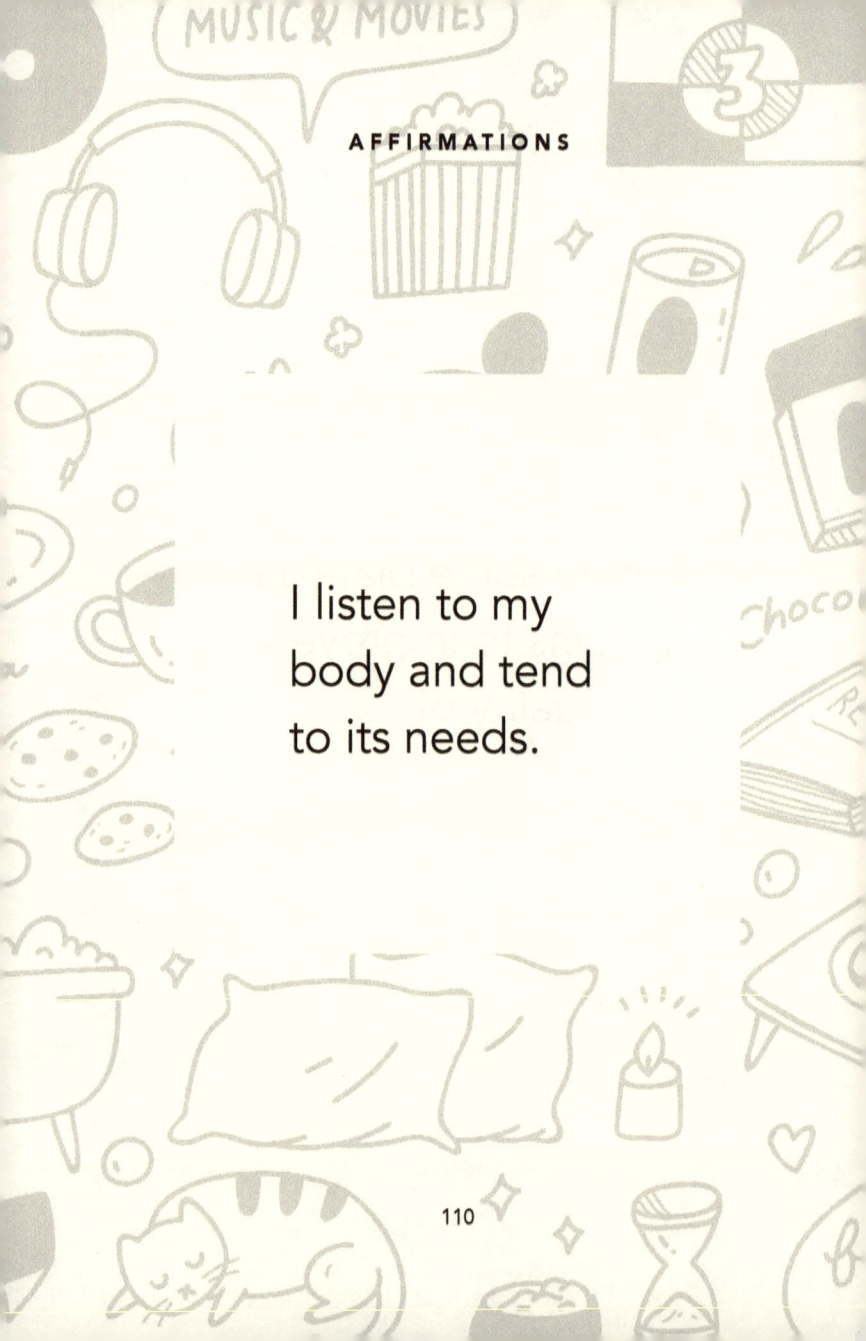

ACTIONS

Re-evaluate your relationships. Ask yourself if it might be time to let go of or stop investing emotionally in those that bring toxicity and negativity into your life.

AFFIRMATIONS

I only get
stronger and
fitter every day.

ACTIONS

The next time a negative thought about yourself pops into your head, imagine saying it to or about someone you love. Chances are, you'll be able to turn that thought right around.

AFFIRMATIONS

I choose to live harmoniously and in perfect balance.

ACTIONS

Look up ways to incorporate essential oils into your day. There are options for a variety of uses, from stress-busting and relaxation to boosting energy.

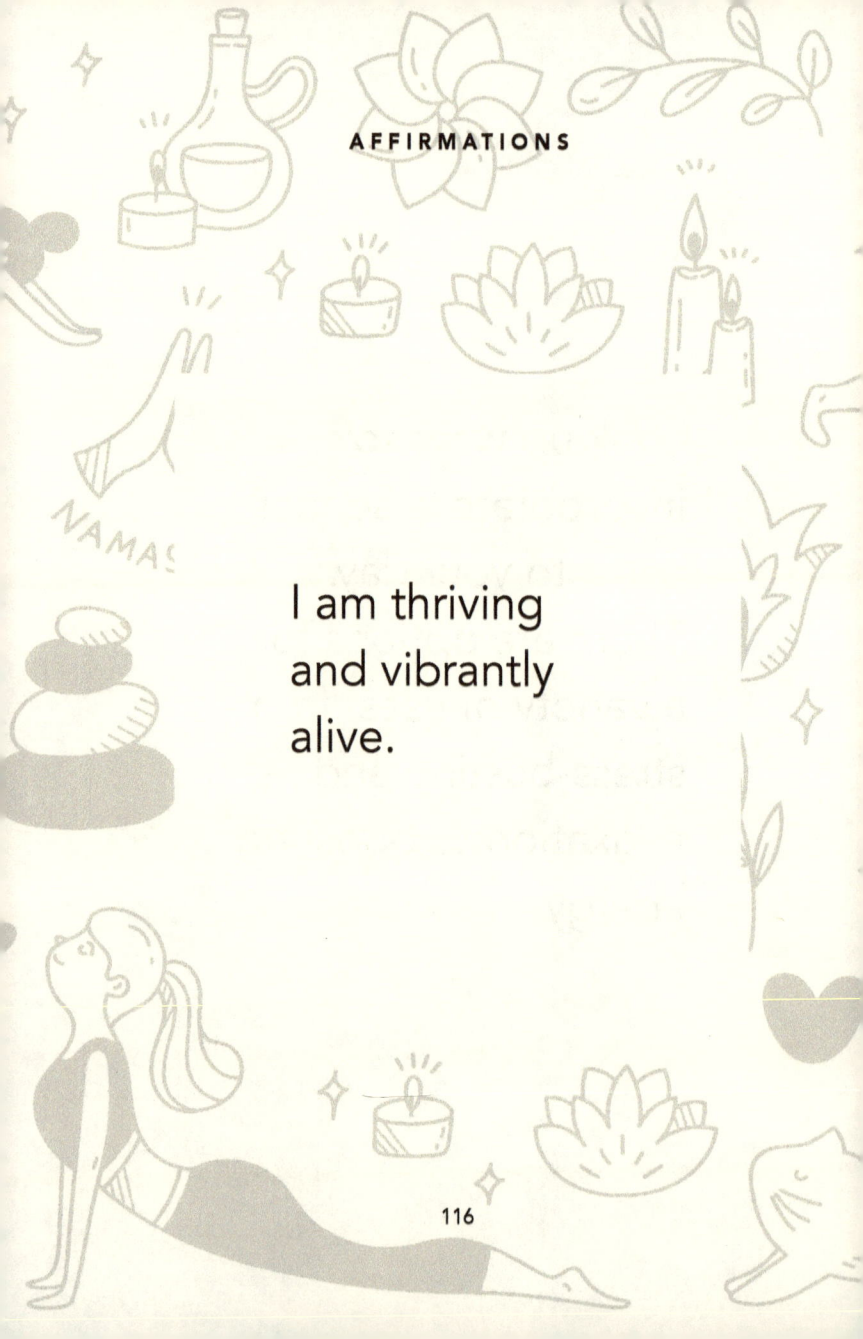

AFFIRMATIONS

I am thriving and vibrantly alive.

ACTIONS

Build a daily journaling habit, taking stock of all aspects of your wellbeing, from physical to emotional.

AFFIRMATIONS

I send my
energy towards
my wellbeing.

ACTIONS

Give yourself permission to say 'no' to something.

AFFIRMATIONS

Every healthy choice I make counts.

ACTIONS

Battle the afternoon slump with a 20-minute power nap.

AFFIRMATIONS

My body loves and supports me.

ACTIONS

Encourage friends and family to join you in your fitness journey!

AFFIRMATIONS

I am in a
constant state
of healing.

ACTIONS

Look into healthy food swaps you can easily, sustainably incorporate into your diet.

AFFIRMATIONS

I have everything it takes to achieve my fittest self.

ACTIONS

Write down 3 things you don't like about yourself. Then, rewrite them into positive, affirming statements.

AFFIRMATIONS

My mind and body are powerfully, wholly connected.

ACTIONS

Stay on top of your annual physical check-ups—when it comes to health, preventive measures go a long way!

AFFIRMATIONS

I am worthy of wellbeing.

ACTIONS

List down 5 things that boost your energy and 5 things that drain it. Take what you learn from this quick exercise into the rest of your week.

AFFIRMATIONS

I allow my
breath to fuel
and move me.

ACTIONS

Stay on track and motivated by joining a fitness community, even just online.

AFFIRMATIONS

I am willing to make healthy changes for myself.

ACTIONS

Replace 2-3 snacks or desserts a week with fruit and veg.

AFFIRMATIONS

I free myself
from any habits
that harm me.

ACTIONS

Once a week, make cooking dinner a family activity!

AFFIRMATIONS

I am fully
committed
to a healthy,
balanced life.

ACTIONS

Create a go-to workout playlist with all your favourite upbeat songs.

AFFIRMATIONS

I deserve rest and recovery.

ACTIONS

Do you have a bad habit you've been meaning to kick? It's time to buckle down and get serious about it—you can do this!

AFFIRMATIONS

I grant my body the grace it needs to grow and flourish in health.

ACTIONS

Set realistic goals and set up sustainable healthy habits. Remember, the journey matters as much (if not more than) the destination.

AFFIRMATIONS

I love how it feels to be active.

ACTIONS

Sign up for a fun run or another physical event you've always wanted to try and commit to training for it.

AFFIRMATIONS

I am not afraid to continue to explore and expand what my body can do.

ACTIONS

Before bed, listen to some ambient sleep sounds like recordings of rain or waves crashing on the beach.

AFFIRMATIONS

I am transforming into the healthiest version of myself.

ACTIONS

Incorporate natural elements such as wood, fresh flowers, or even a small water feature into your indoor space.

AFFIRMATIONS

I cultivate a
healthy mind
and inner self.

ACTIONS

Shake up your fitness routine with a new workout once a week.

Also available by **Kathy Shanks**...

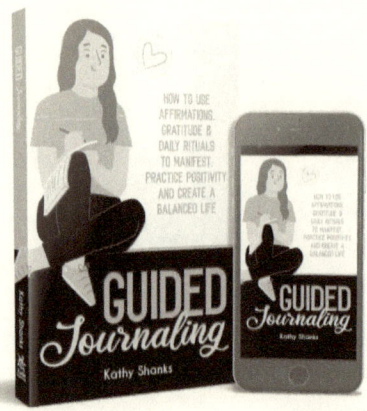

Guided Journaling is available worldwide as print or ebook at Amazon, Booktopia, Barnes & Noble and all good bookstores.

Also available in Australia from **turtlepublishing.com.au**

Inside this book you'll discover how to use my method of journaling to:

- Work towards creating balance for heart, mind, body and soul without sacrificing career and relationships
- Create rituals that help you develop gratitude
- Use daily affirmations to practice positivity and manifest your future dreams
- Discover strategies to improve your relationships, build your life mission, start a side hustle, discover yourself, develop self-love, improve your health AND improve your mindset

It seems too good to be true, right! Organising your thoughts and dreams in 10-20 minutes a day can be that one simple change that actually makes your dreams become a reality.

Make your journal your safe haven, a place of nurturing for you to come and reflect, clear your mind, set goals, develop gratitude, make plans, dream, and take steps towards the future that has always seemed just out of reach.

> Please join our journaling community at
> **facebook.com/groups/kathyshanks**
> for exclusive insider access to updates and releases

Also available in the
Guided Journaling Series...

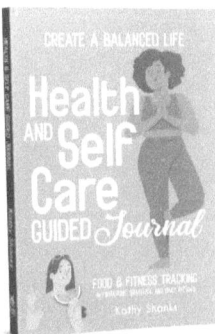

Journaling for a
Balanced Life with a
Health focus

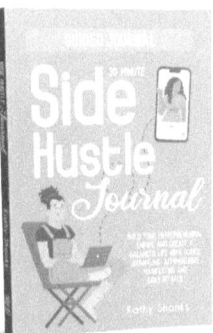

Journaling for a
Balanced Life with a
Life Mission focus

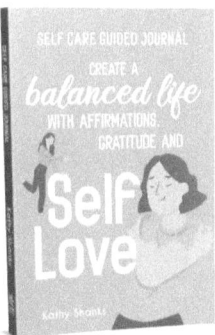

Journaling for a
Balanced Life with a
focus on the **Heart**

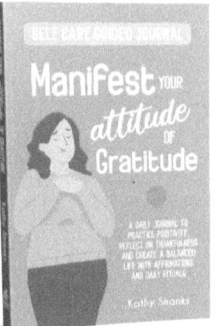

Journaling for a
Balanced Life with a
Gratitude & **Manifest** focus

We have a selection of *journals* available worldwide as
print or ebook at Amazon, Booktopia,
Barnes & Noble and all good bookstores.
Also available in Australia from **turtlepublishing.com.au**

www.ingramcontent.com/pod-product-compliance
Lightning Source LLC
Chambersburg PA
CBHW020323010526
44107CB00054B/1956